NAVIGATING ALZHEIMER'S

A Comprehensive Guide to Understanding, Caring, and Advocating for a Hopeful Future

Dr Philip Ortner

TABLE OF CONTENTS

CHAPTER 1

Introduction to Alzheimer's Disease

Alzheimer's disease (AD) is a complex and challenging condition that affects the brain, gradually impacting memory, thinking abilities, and daily functioning. To better comprehend this condition, we must start by exploring the basics, including its overview, historical context, incidence, prevalence, and a fundamental understanding of the brain and memory function.

Overview of Alzheimer's Disease (AD):

Alzheimer's disease is a progressive neurodegenerative disorder that primarily affects older adults, although it can also occur in individuals as young as their 40s or 50s. It is the most common cause of dementia, a term used to describe a group of symptoms associated with a decline in memory and cognitive abilities. Alzheimer's is a chronic condition, meaning it develops and worsens over time, leading to significant challenges in daily life.

The hallmark of Alzheimer's disease is the accumulation of abnormal protein deposits in the brain. These deposits, called amyloid plaques and neurofibrillary tangles, interfere with the normal functioning of brain cells, ultimately causing them to die. As a result, the communication between brain cells is disrupted, leading to the decline in cognitive abilities.

Historical Context and Discovery:

The story of Alzheimer's disease begins in the early 20th century. In 1906, a German psychiatrist and neuropathologist named Alois Alzheimer made a groundbreaking discovery when he examined the brain tissue of a woman who had experienced severe memory loss, confusion, and personality changes before her death. Under the microscope, he observed the presence of unusual structures in her brain, which later became known as "Alzheimer's plaques" and "neurofibrillary tangles."

This discovery marked a crucial moment in understanding dementia, and over the years, researchers have built upon Alzheimer's work to deepen our knowledge of the disease. The identification of these abnormal protein deposits became a key characteristic of Alzheimer's disease and a focal point for research into its causes and potential treatments.

Incidence and Prevalence

Alzheimer's disease is a widespread and growing health concern worldwide. As societies age and life expectancy increases, the number of people affected by Alzheimer's is on the rise. Statistics reveal that millions of individuals are currently living with Alzheimer's, and the numbers are expected to escalate in the coming years.

The incidence of Alzheimer's refers to the number of new cases diagnosed within a specific time period, while prevalence represents the total number of individuals with the disease at a given point in time. These numbers are influenced by various factors, including age, genetics, and overall population health.

Understanding the incidence and prevalence of Alzheimer's is crucial for public health planning and resource allocation. It helps policymakers, healthcare professionals, and researchers anticipate the growing needs of individuals with Alzheimer's and their families, emphasizing the importance of early diagnosis and effective interventions.

Basic Understanding of the Brain and Memory Function

To comprehend how Alzheimer's disease affects an individual, it's essential to have a basic understanding of the brain and its intricate functions, particularly those related to memory.

The brain is a remarkable organ that controls all bodily functions, enabling us to think, feel, move, and remember. Memory, a fundamental aspect of cognitive function, is a complex process that involves the encoding, storage, and retrieval of information. Different regions of the brain, including the hippocampus and cortex, play vital roles in forming and retrieving memories.

In Alzheimer's disease, these brain regions are progressively damaged, disrupting the normal flow of information and impairing memory function. As the disease advances, individuals may experience difficulties remembering recent events, organizing thoughts, and performing everyday tasks. Understanding this process helps us appreciate the challenges faced by those living with Alzheimer's and provides a foundation for developing supportive strategies and interventions.

CHAPTER 2

Unraveling the Mystery: Causes and Risk Factors

Alzheimer's disease is a complex puzzle, and Chapter 2 delves into the intricate factors that contribute to its development. Understanding the causes and risk factors of Alzheimer's is like peeling back layers of a mystery to reveal the elements that may influence why some individuals are more susceptible to this condition than others.

Genetic Factors and Familial Connections

Genetics plays a significant role in Alzheimer's disease, and researchers have identified specific genes that can influence an individual's susceptibility to the condition. If someone in your family has had Alzheimer's, it might raise concerns about your own risk. Certain genes, such as the APOE gene, have been associated with an increased likelihood of developing Alzheimer's.

However, it's crucial to note that having a family member with Alzheimer's doesn't mean you will definitely get the disease. It simply means there might be a genetic predisposition. Scientists are working hard to understand the intricate interplay between genetics and Alzheimer's, aiming to identify how specific genes contribute to the risk and whether there are ways to mitigate this risk through lifestyle or medical interventions.

Role of Age in Alzheimer's

One of the undeniable factors in Alzheimer's disease is age. The risk of developing Alzheimer's increases as we get older. While Alzheimer's is not a normal part of aging, the likelihood of developing the disease rises significantly after the age of 65. This doesn't mean that everyone over 65 will get Alzheimer's, but the risk does increase with age.

The aging process itself seems to be associated with changes in the brain that make it more vulnerable to diseases like Alzheimer's. As our population ages, the prevalence of Alzheimer's is also on the rise. Understanding the relationship between age and Alzheimer's is vital for healthcare planning and developing strategies to support an aging population.

Lifestyle Factors and Environmental Influences

Beyond genetics and age, our lifestyle choices and the environment we live in also play a crucial role in the development of Alzheimer's disease. Imagine these factors as pieces of the puzzle that, when put together, create a picture of potential risk or protection.

Leading a healthy lifestyle can significantly reduce the risk of Alzheimer's. Regular exercise, a balanced diet, not smoking, and managing conditions like diabetes and hypertension can contribute to overall brain health. Conversely, factors like a sedentary lifestyle, poor diet, smoking, and untreated health conditions can increase the risk.

Environmental influences, such as exposure to toxins or pollutants, are also being explored as potential contributors to Alzheimer's. While the research in this area is ongoing, it highlights the importance of creating environments that support brain health and investigating how external factors might impact our cognitive well-being.

Ongoing Research and Emerging Theories

The mystery of Alzheimer's is far from solved, and scientists around the world are actively engaged in ongoing research to uncover new insights. Chapter 2 provides a glimpse into the cutting-edge investigations and emerging theories that are expanding our understanding of this complex disease.

One exciting area of research involves studying the connections between the brain and other parts of the body, such as the gut. The gut-brain axis is a bidirectional communication system that might play a role in the development of Alzheimer's. Researchers are exploring how the microbiome (the community of microorganisms in our gut) influences brain health and whether interventions targeting the gut could have an impact on Alzheimer's risk.

Another avenue of exploration is the role of inflammation and the immune system in Alzheimer's disease. Chronic inflammation, whether originating in the brain or elsewhere in the body, is being investigated for its potential contribution to the development and progression of Alzheimer's. Understanding these inflammatory processes could open new avenues for treatment and prevention.

CHAPTER 3

The Silent Onset: Recognizing Early Signs

Alzheimer's disease often begins its subtle journey long before it becomes noticeable to the person experiencing it or their loved ones. Chapter 3 explores the crucial topic of recognizing the early signs of Alzheimer's, emphasizing the importance of understanding these subtle changes, differentiating them from normal aging, and the significance of early detection and diagnosis. Through personal stories, this chapter aims to make these concepts relatable and accessible, helping individuals and families navigate the challenging terrain of Alzheimer's onset.

Exploring the Subtle Signs and Symptoms

The early signs of Alzheimer's disease are often quiet whispers rather than loud alarms. Picture it as a gradual dimming of the lights, a slow fading of the vibrant colors of memory and cognition.

Chapter 3 carefully examines these subtle signs and symptoms, such as forgetfulness, difficulty finding the right words, and challenges in planning or solving problems.

Memory loss that disrupts daily life, difficulty completing familiar tasks, confusion with time or place, and changes in mood or personality are some of the early indicators explored in this chapter. It's essential for readers to understand that occasional forgetfulness is a normal part of aging, but persistent and worsening issues may signal something more significant, such as Alzheimer's.

By presenting these signs in relatable terms, the chapter aims to empower readers to recognize potential warning signs in themselves or their loved ones. The goal is to create awareness that prompts proactive engagement with healthcare professionals when needed.

Differentiating Normal Aging from Alzheimer's

As we age, it's common to experience moments of forgetfulness or the occasional struggle to find the right word. However, it's equally important to recognize when these instances cross a threshold into something more concerning. Chapter 3 acts as a guide, providing a framework to differentiate normal aging from potential signs of Alzheimer's disease.

Normal aging might involve misplacing keys or forgetting a name temporarily. In contrast, Alzheimer's-related forgetfulness could involve putting items in unusual places, forgetting names repeatedly, or struggling to complete familiar tasks like cooking a favorite recipe. This chapter aims to clarify these distinctions, offering readers a practical tool to assess whether observed changes align more closely with typical aging or if they warrant further attention.

Understanding these nuances can be a powerful tool for individuals and families, encouraging them to seek professional guidance when needed. Timely intervention can make a significant difference in the management and quality of life for those affected by Alzheimer's.

Importance of Early Detection and Diagnosis

Imagine early detection as a lantern in the darkness—an illumination that allows for informed decisions, access to appropriate support, and the opportunity to engage in treatment and planning. Chapter 3 emphasizes the critical importance of early detection and diagnosis in the context of Alzheimer's disease.

Early diagnosis enables individuals and their families to take proactive steps in managing the condition. It opens doors to available treatments that might help alleviate symptoms and slow down the progression of the disease. Moreover, early detection allows for better planning—financially, legally, and emotionally. It provides an opportunity for individuals to communicate their wishes regarding care and support, ensuring that their preferences are known and respected as the disease progresses.

The chapter also explores the emotional aspects of receiving an Alzheimer's diagnosis. Fear, uncertainty, and a range of emotions often accompany this news. However, understanding that early diagnosis is a tool for empowerment, enabling individuals to navigate their journey with more agency, can be a guiding light in challenging times.

Personal Stories of Individuals Experiencing Early Stages

To make the information in Chapter 3 relatable and human, personal stories take center stage. These narratives provide a window into the lived experiences of individuals in the early stages of Alzheimer's. Readers may find comfort and resonance in these stories, recognizing aspects of their own experiences or those of their loved ones.

By weaving personal stories into the narrative, the chapter aims to reduce stigma and foster empathy. Alzheimer's affects individuals and families in unique ways, and sharing these stories helps demystify the condition. Readers may see aspects of their own journey reflected in the narratives, reinforcing the idea that they are not alone in facing the challenges posed by Alzheimer's disease.

ChaPTER 4

Diagnosis and Assessment

Receiving a diagnosis of Alzheimer's disease is a complex process that involves a series of evaluations and assessments. Chapter 4 delves into this critical aspect, providing a comprehensive understanding of the diagnostic journey. It explores the overview of diagnostic procedures, the role of cognitive assessments and imaging techniques, the emotional impact on individuals and families, and the challenges associated with obtaining an accurate diagnosis.

Overview of Diagnostic Procedures

Imagine a detective carefully gathering clues to solve a mystery. Diagnosing Alzheimer's is somewhat similar—it involves a systematic approach to understanding the symptoms, ruling out other possible causes, and reaching a conclusion based on a combination of evidence.

Chapter 4 opens with an overview of the diagnostic procedures that healthcare professionals use to navigate this intricate process.

First and foremost, a thorough medical history and physical examination are conducted. The doctor will discuss symptoms, lifestyle factors, and any relevant family history. Blood tests may be performed to rule out other conditions that might mimic Alzheimer's symptoms.

Cognitive assessments are a key component of the diagnostic journey. These tests evaluate memory, problem-solving skills, language abilities, and other cognitive functions. They provide valuable information about the extent of cognitive decline and help in establishing a baseline for future comparisons.

Neurological examinations assess factors like reflexes, muscle strength, and coordination. Additionally, brain imaging, such as MRI or CT scans, may be utilized to rule out other potential causes for cognitive decline, like tumors or strokes.

Combining these various pieces of information, healthcare professionals work together like a skilled investigative team, gradually building a comprehensive understanding of the individual's cognitive health.

Cognitive Assessments and Imaging Techniques

Cognitive assessments are akin to snapshots capturing the current state of an individual's cognitive abilities. Chapter 4 delves into the role of these assessments in diagnosing Alzheimer's disease, shedding light on how they help healthcare professionals understand the extent and nature of cognitive decline.

Imagine these assessments as a series of puzzles that, when pieced together, create a detailed picture of cognitive function. The Mini-Mental State Examination (MMSE) is a commonly used tool that assesses various cognitive domains, including memory, attention, and language. The Montreal Cognitive Assessment (MoCA) is another widely used tool that provides a more detailed evaluation of cognitive abilities.

Imaging techniques, such as magnetic resonance imaging (MRI) and positron emission tomography (PET) scans, offer a deeper look into the structure and function of the brain. These images can reveal abnormalities, such as the presence of amyloid plaques and neurofibrillary tangles, which are characteristic of Alzheimer's disease.

While these assessments and imaging techniques are invaluable tools, they are not standalone diagnostic criteria. The collective information from these evaluations contributes to a comprehensive understanding, guiding healthcare professionals in making an accurate diagnosis.

Emotional Impact on Individuals and Families

Receiving a diagnosis of Alzheimer's is not just a medical event; it's a deeply emotional experience that ripples through the lives of individuals and their families. Chapter 4 explores this emotional impact, recognizing the range of feelings—fear, sadness, confusion, and sometimes relief—that accompany the diagnosis.

The emotional impact is not confined to the individual receiving the diagnosis; it extends to family members and caregivers. Learning that a loved one has Alzheimer's can be a heartbreaking revelation, and it often marks the beginning of a profound shift in family dynamics.

Imagine it as a sudden change in the weather—the emotional landscape transforms, and individuals must navigate uncharted territory. Fear of the unknown, grief for the life that was, and the challenges of adapting to a new reality are all part of this emotional journey.

However, it's crucial to recognize that amidst the emotional storm, there can also be moments of resilience, love, and connection. Chapter 4 seeks to offer support and understanding to individuals and families navigating the emotional terrain of an Alzheimer's diagnosis. It emphasizes the importance of seeking help from support groups, mental health professionals, and other resources to cope with the emotional challenges.

Challenges in Obtaining an Accurate Diagnosis

Diagnosing Alzheimer's disease is a nuanced process, and Chapter 4 addresses the challenges associated with obtaining an accurate diagnosis. The complexity of Alzheimer's, the overlap of symptoms with other conditions, and variations in individual experiences all contribute to the diagnostic challenges.

Imagine trying to solve a puzzle with missing pieces. In the case of Alzheimer's, the puzzle pieces might be elusive, and some symptoms may overlap with those of other conditions, such as depression or certain vitamin deficiencies. Additionally, individuals may downplay their symptoms or be unaware of the extent of their cognitive decline, posing challenges for accurate reporting during assessments.

The chapter sheds light on the importance of a multidisciplinary approach, where healthcare professionals collaborate and consider a range of factors to arrive at a comprehensive diagnosis. It also emphasizes the need for ongoing monitoring and reevaluation, as Alzheimer's is a dynamic condition with symptoms that may evolve over time.

CHAPTER 5

Beyond Memory: Understanding Behavioral Changes

Alzheimer's disease not only affects memory but also introduces a range of behavioral and psychological symptoms that can significantly impact the daily lives of individuals and their relationships. Chapter 5 delves into this multifaceted aspect of Alzheimer's, exploring the Behavioral and Psychological Symptoms of Dementia (BPSD), examining their impact on daily life and relationships, providing strategies for coping with challenging behaviors, and highlighting the crucial support needed for caregivers and family members.

Behavioral and Psychological Symptoms of Dementia (BPSD)

Imagine Alzheimer's disease as a painter, creating a canvas of challenges that extend beyond memory loss. BPSD, or Behavioral and Psychological

Symptoms of Dementia, are the various colors on this canvas. These symptoms encompass a broad range of behaviors and emotional experiences that individuals with Alzheimer's may exhibit.

Common BPSD include agitation, aggression, anxiety, depression, hallucinations, delusions, and sleep disturbances. It's crucial to understand that these symptoms are often expressions of underlying issues, such as confusion, frustration, or unmet needs. Chapter 5 begins by unraveling the complexities of BPSD, helping readers see beyond the surface behaviors to understand the emotions and experiences driving them.

Impact on Daily Life and Relationships

BPSD can cast a shadow over daily life, altering routines and challenging the dynamics of relationships. Imagine the familiar paths of daily activities now filled with unpredictable twists and turns. For example, agitation or aggression may disrupt routine tasks, and sleep disturbances can lead to exhaustion for both the individual with Alzheimer's and their caregivers.

This chapter delves into the day-to-day challenges that families and caregivers face, emphasizing the need for flexibility and understanding. The impact on relationships can be profound, as individuals with Alzheimer's may struggle to communicate their needs or express their emotions. This can lead to frustration, confusion, and strained interactions.

The goal of this section is to humanize the experience, acknowledging the difficulties faced by individuals and their loved ones while offering insights into how to navigate these challenges with compassion and resilience. It emphasizes the importance of adapting expectations and finding new ways to connect and communicate.

Strategies for Coping with Challenging Behaviors

Navigating the behavioral changes associated with Alzheimer's requires a toolkit of strategies that caregivers and family members can use to promote a positive and supportive environment. Imagine these strategies as the compass and map for a journey through unfamiliar terrain.

One essential strategy is effective communication. Picture communication as a dance where verbal and nonverbal cues play a significant role. Patience, active listening, and a calm demeanor become essential steps in this dance, helping individuals with Alzheimer's feel understood and supported.

Creating a structured and familiar environment is another valuable strategy. Consistent routines, clear signage, and a clutter-free space can provide a sense of security and reduce confusion. This chapter explores these and other practical strategies, offering readers a repertoire of approaches to address specific behaviors associated with Alzheimer's.

Additionally, the importance of addressing the root causes of behaviors is highlighted. Understanding that BPSD often signal unmet needs—such as pain, hunger, or the need for social interaction—guides caregivers in responding with empathy and problem-solving.

Support for Caregivers and Family Members

Caring for someone with Alzheimer's is a demanding and emotionally challenging role. Picture caregivers as the unsung heroes, navigating the twists and turns of the Alzheimer's journey with dedication and love. Chapter 5 recognizes the vital role of caregivers and family members, emphasizing the need for a robust support system.

Caregivers often face physical, emotional, and financial strain. The chapter explores the importance of seeking support from healthcare professionals, support groups, and community resources. Just as a team supports each other in a relay race, caregivers need a network of support to share the responsibilities and alleviate the burden.

Respite care is also discussed as a crucial aspect of caregiver support. Picture it as a moment of rest during a marathon—essential for recharging physical and emotional reserves. Respite care allows caregivers to take a break, attend to their own needs, and return to their caregiving role with renewed energy.

Moreover, the chapter emphasizes the significance of maintaining open communication within families. Discussing the challenges, sharing feelings, and working together as a team create a more supportive environment for both the individual with Alzheimer's and their caregivers.

CHAPTER 6

Living with Alzheimer's: Navigating Daily Challenges

Living with Alzheimer's presents a unique set of daily challenges, not only for the individual with the condition but also for their caregivers and family members. Chapter 6 delves into practical aspects of day-to-day life, offering adaptive strategies for daily activities, exploring home modifications and safety considerations, addressing legal and financial planning, and highlighting the support services and resources available to individuals and families on this journey.

Adaptive Strategies for Daily Activities

Imagine daily activities as a series of interconnected puzzles. For individuals with Alzheimer's, these puzzles may become more challenging, requiring creative solutions and adaptive strategies. Chapter 6 begins by exploring how to approach daily activities with flexibility and ingenuity.

Adaptive strategies involve simplifying tasks, breaking them into smaller steps, and utilizing cues to guide the individual through the process. Picture it as creating a roadmap with clear signs for each step of the journey. For example, labeling drawers or using color-coded cues can help in organizing and finding items.

Establishing routines becomes a cornerstone of daily life. Routines offer predictability and a sense of security, reducing anxiety for individuals with Alzheimer's. This chapter provides insights into creating structured routines for various activities, fostering a sense of accomplishment and independence.

Moreover, the chapter addresses communication strategies. Imagine communication as a dance where verbal and nonverbal cues play significant roles. Using clear and simple language, maintaining eye contact, and practicing patience become essential steps in this dance, promoting effective communication and understanding.

Home Modifications and Safety Considerations

Transforming a living space into a safe and supportive environment is a critical aspect of living with Alzheimer's. Chapter 6 explores home modifications and safety considerations, envisioning the home as a haven that balances independence with safety.

Imagine the home as a carefully curated exhibit where each element contributes to a supportive and secure atmosphere. Simple modifications, such as removing trip hazards, installing grab bars, and improving lighting, can significantly enhance safety. The chapter provides practical guidance on making these modifications, ensuring that the living space adapts to the changing needs of the individual with Alzheimer's.

Addressing wandering behavior, a common concern in Alzheimer's, involves implementing additional safety measures. Picture it as creating a secure perimeter within the home or utilizing technology, such as door alarms, to prevent unintended exits. The goal is to strike a balance between fostering independence and ensuring safety.

Moreover, the chapter explores considerations for bedroom safety, emphasizing the importance of a comfortable and secure sleep environment. Creating a calming bedtime routine and ensuring that the bedroom is free from potential hazards contribute to a restful night's sleep.

Legal and Financial Planning

Navigating the legal and financial aspects of living with Alzheimer's requires thoughtful planning and foresight. Chapter 6 envisions legal and financial planning as a roadmap, guiding individuals and their families through the complexities of future decision-making.

Legal planning involves creating essential documents, such as a power of attorney and advance directives. Imagine these documents as shields, offering protection and guidance when important decisions need to be made. The chapter provides insights into the importance of appointing trusted individuals to make financial and healthcare decisions on behalf of the individual with Alzheimer's.

Financial planning encompasses budgeting, managing assets, and exploring available resources. Picture it as constructing a sturdy foundation that supports the individual's current and future needs. The chapter explores strategies for financial planning, including consulting with financial professionals, identifying available benefits, and understanding long-term care options.

Long-term care planning becomes a focal point, envisioning a future where the individual's care needs are met with dignity and respect. The chapter provides information on the different types of long-term care, such as in-home care and assisted living, helping individuals and their families make informed decisions based on their unique circumstances.

Support Services and Resources Available for Individuals and Families:

Living with Alzheimer's is a journey that benefits from a strong support network. Chapter 6 envisions support services and resources as a vast landscape of assistance, offering guidance and companionship throughout the Alzheimer's experience.

Imagine a support network as a community of individuals and organizations working together to provide assistance. The chapter explores various support services, such as caregiver support groups, respite care, and adult day programs, offering caregivers opportunities to connect with others facing similar challenges.

Community resources, such as senior centers and local organizations, become pillars of support. Picture them as hubs of information and assistance, offering educational programs, social activities, and practical help for individuals and their families.

Moreover, the chapter highlights the role of healthcare professionals in the support network. Envision healthcare professionals as guides, offering expertise and personalized care plans to address the unique needs of individuals with Alzheimer's. Regular check-ups, medication management, and collaboration with specialists contribute to comprehensive healthcare support.

CHAPTER 7

Medications and Therapies

Living with Alzheimer's disease often involves a journey through the landscape of medications and therapies aimed at managing symptoms and potentially slowing the progression of the disease. Chapter 7 delves into this complex terrain, providing an overview of available medications, exploring their potential benefits and limitations, discussing emerging therapies and research advancements, and highlighting the importance of personalized treatment plans.

Overview of Available Medications

Imagine medications as tools in a toolbox, each serving a specific purpose in managing the challenges of Alzheimer's disease. Chapter 7 opens with an overview of the medications commonly prescribed to address cognitive symptoms and enhance quality of life for individuals with Alzheimer's.

Cholinesterase inhibitors, such as donepezil, rivastigmine, and galantamine, are often prescribed to boost levels of a neurotransmitter called acetylcholine. Picture acetylcholine as a messenger facilitating communication between brain cells. These medications aim to enhance this communication, temporarily alleviating some cognitive symptoms.

Another class of medications, NMDA receptor antagonists like memantine, works by regulating the activity of another neurotransmitter, glutamate. Imagine glutamate as the conductor of an orchestra, influencing brain cell communication. Memantine helps modulate this communication, providing additional support for cognitive function.

These medications don't cure Alzheimer's, but they can help manage symptoms, providing individuals and their families with a measure of stability and improved quality of life.

Potential Benefits and Limitations

Understanding the potential benefits and limitations of medications for Alzheimer's is crucial. Picture the benefits as patches of sunlight breaking through the clouds—providing moments of relief and improved functioning. However, it's equally important to acknowledge the limitations, represented by the persistent clouds that cannot be entirely dispelled.

The benefits of medications include improvements in cognitive function, enhanced ability to perform daily activities, and potentially a slower progression of symptoms. Individuals may experience increased alertness, better communication, and a more stable mood, contributing to an improved overall quality of life.

However, these medications are not a cure, and their effects vary from person to person. Some individuals may experience significant benefits, while others may see only modest improvements or none at all. It's essential to manage expectations and recognize that medications may not halt the progression of the disease.

Moreover, medications may come with side effects, ranging from mild to more severe. Picture side effects as occasional storms that accompany patches of sunlight. These side effects can include nausea, diarrhea, insomnia, and muscle cramps. The chapter delves into the importance of open communication with healthcare professionals to monitor and manage potential side effects, ensuring that the benefits outweigh any drawbacks.

Emerging Therapies and Research Advancements

Imagine the field of Alzheimer's research as a garden of possibilities, with scientists and researchers cultivating new ideas and approaches to understand and treat the disease. Chapter 7 explores emerging therapies and research advancements, envisioning a future where innovative treatments offer hope for individuals with Alzheimer's.

One area of active research involves anti-amyloid and anti-tau therapies. Amyloid plaques and tau tangles are abnormal protein deposits in the brain associated with Alzheimer's. Emerging therapies aim to prevent the formation of these deposits or clear them from the brain, potentially slowing the disease's progression.

Immunotherapy is another promising avenue. Picture it as strengthening the body's defenses against Alzheimer's-related proteins.

Immunotherapies stimulate the immune system to recognize and remove these proteins, offering a targeted approach to address the underlying causes of the disease.

Lifestyle interventions, including diet, exercise, and cognitive stimulation, are also under investigation. Imagine these interventions as seeds planted in the garden of well-being, contributing to overall brain health and potentially reducing the risk of Alzheimer's.

Clinical trials play a pivotal role in advancing research. Envision clinical trials as pathways through the garden, testing the effectiveness and safety of new treatments. Chapter 7 encourages individuals and their families to consider participation in clinical trials, recognizing the importance of collective efforts to unlock new possibilities in Alzheimer's treatment.

The Importance of Personalized Treatment Plans

In the realm of Alzheimer's medications and therapies, one size does not fit all. Chapter 7 underscores the importance of personalized treatment plans, envisioning them as tailored garments designed to address the unique needs and circumstances of each individual with Alzheimer's.

Personalized treatment plans consider factors such as age, overall health, coexisting conditions, and individual responses to medications. Imagine these plans as dynamic and flexible, adjusting to the changing needs of the individual as Alzheimer's progresses.

Communication between healthcare professionals, individuals with Alzheimer's, and their families becomes a cornerstone of personalized treatment. Picture it as a collaborative effort, with everyone working together to understand the individual's experiences, preferences, and goals.

Moreover, the chapter highlights the significance of regular follow-ups and adjustments to treatment plans. Imagine this process as fine-tuning, ensuring that the medications and therapies continue to align with the individual's evolving needs and circumstances.

CHAPTER 8

Caregiving: Balancing Love and Responsibility

Caregiving for a loved one with Alzheimer's disease is a profound journey marked by love, responsibility, and the delicate balance between meeting the needs of the individual and maintaining the well-being of the caregiver. Chapter 8 delves into the intricate world of caregiving, exploring the emotional and physical toll on caregivers, emphasizing the importance of building a support network, discussing the necessity of self-care, and addressing the challenges of coping with grief and loss along the caregiving journey.

Emotional and Physical Toll on Caregivers:

Imagine the role of a caregiver as a sturdy bridge, connecting the individual with Alzheimer's to a world of care and support. This bridge, however, is not without its challenges. Chapter 8 opens by acknowledging the emotional and physical toll that caregiving can take on individuals who selflessly dedicate themselves to the well-being of their loved ones.

The emotional toll often manifests as stress, anxiety, and a range of complex emotions. Picture it as a storm brewing within, where caregivers navigate the turbulent waters of uncertainty and the challenges presented by Alzheimer's. The chapter explores the emotional landscape, offering insights into the various feelings that caregivers may experience, including guilt, frustration, and sadness.

The physical toll is akin to the wear and tear on the bridge's structure. Caregiving can lead to exhaustion, sleep disturbances, and compromised physical health. Picture it as the weight of responsibility taking its toll on the caregiver's well-being. The chapter delves into the importance of recognizing and addressing both the emotional and physical aspects of caregiving, emphasizing that caring for oneself is an essential component of effective caregiving.

Building a Support Network

In the vast terrain of caregiving, a support network becomes the compass, guiding caregivers through the challenges and providing a sense of direction. Chapter 8 envisions a support network as a circle of care, recognizing the interconnected relationships that sustain and uplift caregivers.

Family members, friends, and neighbors form the inner circle of this support network. Picture them as pillars of strength, offering assistance with daily tasks, providing emotional support, and creating a sense of community. The chapter explores strategies for building and maintaining these crucial connections, fostering an environment where caregivers feel seen, heard, and understood.

Professional support, including healthcare professionals, support groups, and social services, becomes the outer circle of the support network. Imagine these professionals as guides, offering expertise, information, and a broader perspective on caregiving challenges. The chapter encourages caregivers to tap into these resources, recognizing that seeking help is not a sign of weakness but a testament to strength and resilience.

Additionally, technology can be a valuable ally in building a support network. Picture it as a bridge that spans distances, connecting caregivers to online communities, telehealth services, and information resources. The chapter explores the role of technology in facilitating communication, accessing information, and promoting a sense of belonging within the broader caregiving community.

Self-Care for Caregivers

In the whirlwind of caregiving responsibilities, self-care becomes a lifeboat—a crucial means of navigating the challenges while ensuring the caregiver's own well-being. Chapter 8 envisions self-care as a compass, guiding caregivers to prioritize their physical, emotional, and mental health.

Physical self-care involves simple yet impactful practices, such as maintaining a healthy diet, getting regular exercise, and ensuring adequate rest. Picture it as tending to the bridge's foundational structure, strengthening it to withstand the demands of caregiving.

Emotional self-care is like the bridge's support cables, providing stability and resilience. The chapter explores mindfulness techniques, relaxation exercises, and ways to express and process emotions. Caregivers are encouraged to acknowledge their feelings, seek emotional outlets, and engage in activities that bring joy and fulfillment.

Mental self-care is akin to regularly inspecting and maintaining the bridge's components. Caregivers are encouraged to stimulate their minds through activities such as reading, puzzles, or engaging in hobbies. Seeking opportunities for learning and personal growth contributes to mental well-being.

The chapter emphasizes that self-care is not a luxury but a necessity, reminding caregivers that taking care of themselves allows them to be more effective and present in their caregiving role. It envisions self-care as a continuous practice, woven into the fabric of daily life.

Coping with Grief and Loss In the Caregiving Journey

The caregiving journey is marked by moments of joy, connection, and love, but it is also accompanied by grief and loss. Chapter 8 acknowledges that grief is an integral part of the caregiving landscape, envisioning it as a river that caregivers navigate, with its ebbs and flows.

Grief may manifest at various points in the caregiving journey, from the initial diagnosis to witnessing the progression of Alzheimer's. Picture it as the changing landscape along the riverbanks, where caregivers grapple with the loss of the person they once knew and the evolving nature of their relationship.

Anticipatory grief, the mourning that occurs before a loss, is a significant aspect of caregiving. The chapter explores this concept, recognizing that caregivers may experience a range of emotions as they anticipate and adjust to the changes in their loved one's abilities and personality.

Moreover, the chapter discusses the grieving process after the passing of a loved one, envisioning it as a tributary that flows into the main river of grief. Caregivers are encouraged to allow themselves time and space to mourn, seek support from their network, and explore avenues for grief counseling if needed.

CHAPTER 9

Advocacy and Awareness

Advocacy and awareness form the heartbeat of the collective effort to understand, support, and find solutions for Alzheimer's disease. Chapter 9 delves into the crucial role of advocacy in Alzheimer's research and support, the importance of breaking down stigma and misconceptions, strategies for promoting community awareness and understanding, and the significance of individuals participating in clinical trials and research studies. In this chapter, envision Alzheimer's advocacy as a force that drives change, dispels myths, and fosters a community dedicated to making a difference.

The Role of Advocacy in Alzheimer's Research and Support

Advocacy is the engine that propels progress in Alzheimer's research and support. Picture it as a team of dedicated individuals pushing a boulder uphill, overcoming obstacles to advance our understanding of the disease and improve the lives of those affected.

In the realm of research, advocates play a vital role in urging for increased funding, policy changes, and support for innovative approaches. The chapter envisions these advocates as voices that echo in legislative halls, advocating for resources and policies that prioritize Alzheimer's research. Their efforts contribute to breakthroughs, advancements in treatment options, and a deeper understanding of the disease.

Advocacy extends beyond research to support services and resources for individuals living with Alzheimer's and their caregivers. Imagine it as a network of support, ensuring that those affected by the disease have access to the care, information, and assistance they need. Advocates work to shape healthcare policies, promote caregiver support programs, and enhance the quality of life for those on the Alzheimer's journey.

The chapter emphasizes that advocacy is not confined to large-scale efforts; even individual voices contribute to the collective impact. Advocacy involves raising awareness, sharing personal stories, and engaging with policymakers to create a supportive environment for those affected by Alzheimer's.

Breaking Down Stigma and Misconceptions

Stigma surrounding Alzheimer's disease can be a formidable barrier, preventing individuals from seeking help, accessing support, and understanding the complexities of the condition. Chapter 9 envisions advocates as myth busters, dispelling misconceptions and fostering a more compassionate and informed community.

Imagine stigma as a dark cloud hanging over the Alzheimer's experience. Advocates work to break through this cloud, challenging stereotypes and promoting a more accurate understanding of the disease. They highlight that Alzheimer's is not a normal part of aging but a medical condition that deserves empathy, support, and research attention.

Advocates also address misconceptions about the abilities and worth of individuals living with Alzheimer's. Picture it as unveiling the hidden talents and strengths that persist despite cognitive decline. By showcasing the resilience and unique qualities of individuals with Alzheimer's, advocates contribute to reshaping public perceptions.

Moreover, the chapter explores the impact of language in breaking down stigma. Imagine language as a bridge that connects individuals, fostering understanding and empathy. Advocates encourage the use of person-centered language that respects the dignity of those with Alzheimer's, emphasizing the person behind the diagnosis rather than defining them by their condition.

Promoting Community Awareness and Understanding:

Creating a community that is aware, understanding, and supportive of Alzheimer's is a shared responsibility. Chapter 9 envisions advocates as architects, designing a foundation of knowledge and empathy that transforms communities into spaces where individuals with Alzheimer's can live with dignity and inclusion.

Community awareness involves reaching beyond the immediate circles of those directly affected by Alzheimer's. Picture it as ripples spreading across a pond, gradually expanding the reach of understanding and support. Advocates engage with schools, workplaces, and community organizations, offering educational programs, raising awareness, and fostering a culture of empathy.

One key aspect of promoting understanding is providing information about the early signs of Alzheimer's and the importance of early diagnosis. Imagine it as planting seeds of knowledge, empowering individuals to recognize potential symptoms, seek help, and navigate the complexities of the disease with a proactive mindset.

Support groups and community events become hubs of awareness and understanding. Picture them as gathering places where individuals can share their experiences, ask questions, and find solace in the company of others facing similar challenges. Advocates work to establish and promote these support networks, recognizing their role in reducing isolation and fostering a sense of community.

Participating in Clinical Trials and Research Studies

Participating in clinical trials and research studies is akin to joining an expedition—an opportunity for individuals to contribute to the exploration of new frontiers in Alzheimer's research. Chapter 9 envisions advocates as pioneers, encouraging individuals to play an active role in advancing our understanding of the disease and testing innovative treatments.

Clinical trials are the laboratories where potential breakthroughs are tested and refined. Imagine them as fields where researchers plant seeds of discovery, with participants as essential contributors to the growth of knowledge. Advocates work to dispel fears and misconceptions surrounding clinical trials, emphasizing their importance in advancing Alzheimer's research.

The chapter explores the benefits and considerations of participating in clinical trials.

Picture it as a decision-making compass, guiding individuals through the process of weighing potential risks and benefits. Advocates encourage informed decision-making, emphasizing that participation in research is a valuable contribution to the broader Alzheimer's community.

Moreover, the chapter highlights the role of research registries as bridges that connect individuals interested in participating in studies with researchers seeking participants. These registries envision a future where a diverse range of voices contributes to research, ensuring that findings are relevant and applicable to the broader population.

CHAPTER 10

The Future of Alzheimer's: Hope and Progress

As we peer into the future of Alzheimer's, Chapter 10 unfolds like a tapestry, weaving together threads of promising research, potential breakthroughs, advances in technology and treatment approaches, the importance of a holistic approach to care, and encouraging messages of hope and resilience. Envision this chapter as a compass pointing toward a future where progress transforms the landscape of Alzheimer's, offering not only innovative solutions but also a vision of hope for individuals and families affected by the disease.

Promising Research and Potential Breakthroughs

The future of Alzheimer's is illuminated by the beacon of research—a dynamic and evolving field where scientists, clinicians, and advocates collaborate to unravel the mysteries of the disease.

Picture research as a series of doors, each potentially leading to breakthroughs that could change the trajectory of Alzheimer's.

One avenue of research focuses on understanding and targeting the underlying biological processes of the disease. Imagine it as deciphering a complex code—the genetic, molecular, and cellular intricacies that contribute to Alzheimer's. Researchers explore therapies that target abnormal protein deposits, such as beta-amyloid plaques and tau tangles, with the hope of slowing or halting disease progression.

Another promising area involves exploring the role of inflammation and the immune system in Alzheimer's. Picture it as uncovering the body's defense mechanisms, with researchers investigating ways to modulate the immune response to mitigate the impact of the disease.

In the realm of drug development, envision a diverse array of compounds being tested for their potential to alter the course of Alzheimer's. Researchers are exploring new medications that target different aspects of brain function, aiming to improve cognition, enhance memory, and address behavioral symptoms.

Clinical trials become the testing grounds for these potential breakthroughs. Picture them as bridges between research discoveries and real-world applications. The future holds the promise of individuals with Alzheimer's having access to treatments that not only manage symptoms but also target the underlying causes of the disease.

Advances in Technology and Treatment Approaches

Technology emerges as a key player in shaping the future of Alzheimer's care and treatment. Envision it as a toolbox filled with innovative solutions that enhance diagnosis, improve daily life, and provide support for individuals with Alzheimer's and their caregivers.

Diagnostic tools are advancing, offering more accurate and accessible methods for detecting Alzheimer's in its early stages. Imagine these tools as precision instruments, allowing healthcare professionals to identify the disease before significant cognitive decline occurs. Early diagnosis opens the door to timely interventions and personalized treatment plans.

Telehealth becomes a transformative force, especially for individuals living in remote areas or facing mobility challenges. Picture it as a virtual bridge connecting individuals with Alzheimer's to healthcare professionals, support services, and educational resources. Telehealth facilitates regular check-ups, medication management, and access to valuable information for both individuals and their caregivers.

Technology also plays a role in enhancing daily life for individuals with Alzheimer's. Imagine apps and devices as navigational aids, providing prompts for daily tasks, medication reminders, and cognitive stimulation. These tools contribute to a more supportive and adaptive environment, fostering independence and quality of life.

In the realm of treatment approaches, envision a shift toward personalized and holistic care. Picture it as a departure from one-size-fits-all solutions to tailored interventions that consider the unique needs, preferences, and circumstances of each individual. Integrative approaches encompass a combination of medications, lifestyle interventions, and support services that address the physical, emotional, and cognitive aspects of Alzheimer's.

The Importance of a Holistic Approach to Care

The future of Alzheimer's care embraces a holistic approach that recognizes the interconnected aspects of an individual's well-being. Imagine care as a tapestry, woven with threads of medical, emotional, and social support that collectively contribute to a comprehensive and compassionate approach.

Medical care involves not only addressing cognitive symptoms but also managing coexisting conditions and promoting overall health. Picture it as a collaborative effort between healthcare professionals, individuals with Alzheimer's, and their caregivers to create personalized care plans that prioritize well-being.

Emotional and social support form essential components of the holistic approach. Envision them as pillars that provide stability and comfort, recognizing the emotional toll of Alzheimer's on individuals and their caregivers. Support groups, counseling services, and community resources become integral to creating a network of understanding and empathy.

Lifestyle interventions contribute to the holistic approach by emphasizing the importance of diet, exercise, and cognitive stimulation. Picture them as elements of a well-balanced routine that promotes physical health, cognitive function, and emotional resilience. Care plans include strategies for maintaining a healthy lifestyle, fostering a sense of purpose and engagement.

Moreover, the holistic approach extends to caregiver support. Imagine it as a recognition of the crucial role caregivers play in the Alzheimer's journey. Support services, respite care, and education become integral components of care plans, acknowledging the well-being of caregivers and their essential contribution to the overall care ecosystem.

Encouraging Messages of Hope and Resilience

As we look to the future, envision a landscape illuminated by messages of hope and resilience. Picture these messages as beacons of light, inspiring individuals and families affected by Alzheimer's to navigate the challenges with strength and optimism.

Hope is embedded in the progress of research and the development of innovative treatments. Imagine it as a sunrise, signaling the dawn of new possibilities and a brighter future for those living with Alzheimer's. Messages of hope emphasize that, even in the face of a challenging disease, there are reasons to believe in the potential for positive change.

Resilience becomes a guiding principle for individuals and caregivers alike. Envision it as a sturdy bridge that withstands the winds of adversity, allowing individuals with Alzheimer's and their caregivers to adapt, learn, and find strength in the midst of challenges. Messages of resilience highlight the power of the human spirit and the capacity to forge a meaningful and fulfilling life despite the impact of Alzheimer's.

Community support and awareness contribute to the messages of hope and resilience. Picture them as a chorus of voices that uplift and encourage. Advocacy efforts and increased public understanding foster a sense of solidarity, reminding individuals and families that they are not alone in their Alzheimer's journey.

CONCLUSION

In concluding the exploration of Alzheimer's disease across the ten chapters, we have embarked on a comprehensive journey through the various facets of this complex condition. Each chapter, like a distinct chapter in a book, has unfolded the layers of Alzheimer's, from its historical context and early signs to diagnosis, caregiving, advocacy, and a hopeful look into the future. Let's summarize the key takeaways from our exploration.

Understanding Alzheimer's

Alzheimer's disease is more than a medical condition; it is a journey that impacts individuals, families, and communities. The journey begins with an understanding of Alzheimer's as a progressive neurodegenerative disorder that primarily affects memory, cognition, and daily functioning.

The Journey through Alzheimer's

1. **Introduction to Alzheimer's (Chapter 1):** Explored the basics of Alzheimer's, its historical context, prevalence, and the fundamental understanding of the brain and memory function.

2. **Causes and Risk Factors (Chapter 2):** Dived into the genetic, age-related, and lifestyle factors contributing to Alzheimer's, along with ongoing research and emerging theories.

3. **Recognizing Early Signs (Chapter 3):** Explored the subtle symptoms of Alzheimer's, differentiating them from normal aging, and stressed the importance of early detection.

4. **Diagnosis and Assessment (Chapter 4):** Discussed the diagnostic procedures, cognitive assessments, emotional impact,

and challenges in obtaining an accurate diagnosis.

5. **Understanding Behavioral Changes (Chapter 5):** Examined the behavioral and psychological symptoms of dementia, their impact, coping strategies, and support for caregivers.

6. **Living with Alzheimer's (Chapter 6):** Explored adaptive strategies for daily activities, home modifications, legal and financial planning, and the support services available for individuals and families.

7. **Medications and Therapies (Chapter 7):** Unveiled the available medications, their benefits and limitations, emerging therapies, and the importance of personalized treatment plans.

8. **Caregiving (Chapter 8):** Addressed the emotional and physical toll on caregivers, the importance of building a support

network, self-care practices, and coping with grief and loss.

9. **Advocacy and Awareness (Chapter 9):** Explored the role of advocacy in research and support, breaking down stigma, promoting community awareness, and the significance of participating in clinical trials.

10. **The Future of Alzheimer's (Chapter 10):** Envisioned a future marked by promising research, technological advances, holistic care approaches, and encouraging messages of hope and resilience.

Key Themes

- **Holistic Approach:** Emphasized the importance of a holistic approach to Alzheimer's care, recognizing the interconnected aspects of physical, emotional, and social well-being.

- **Advocacy and Awareness:** Explored the pivotal role of advocacy in advancing research, breaking down stigma, and fostering community understanding. Advocacy serves as a powerful force for change in the Alzheimer's landscape.

- **Hope and Resilience:** Concluded with a vision of hope for the future, highlighting promising research, technological advancements, and messages of resilience that inspire individuals and families affected by Alzheimer's.

In essence, the exploration of Alzheimer's has been a journey of understanding, empathy, and empowerment. It is a journey that acknowledges the challenges but also celebrates the resilience of individuals facing Alzheimer's and the strength of the communities that support them. As we navigate the complexities of Alzheimer's, the overarching theme remains one of compassion—a shared commitment to enhancing the quality of life for those affected by Alzheimer's and collectively working toward a future where the journey is marked by progress, understanding, and hope.

www.ingramcontent.com/pod-product-compliance
Lightning Source LLC
Chambersburg PA
CBHW050743260726
48661CB00001B/393